Contents

What is pancreatitis?

Pancreatitis is a serious condition that occurs when the pancreas becomes inflamed. The pancreas is an organ that produces insulin and digestive enzymes. The same enzymes that help with digestion can sometimes injure the pancreas and cause irritation. This irritation can be short-term or long-term.

There are two forms of pancreatitis:

• Acute pancreatitis is a sudden and short bout of inflammation.

• Chronic pancreatitis is ongoing inflammation.

Where is the pancreas located?

The pancreas is an organ in the upper abdomen (belly). It connects to the beginning of the small intestine (the duodenum). It contains the pancreatic duct (tube), which drains digestive enzymes (chemicals) into the small intestine (the duodenum).

What is the function of the pancreas?

Your pancreas has two primary functions. First, it makes digestive enzymes (chemicals) and releases them into the small intestine. These enzymes break down carbohydrates, proteins and fat from food.

Your pancreas also produces several hormones and releases them into the blood. Amongst these hormones is insulin which regulates the amount of sugar in your blood (glucose). Insulin also helps provide energy now and stores some for later.

Who gets pancreatitis?

You're more likely to develop pancreatitis if you:

• Are male.

• Are African-American.

• Have other people in your family who've had pancreatitis.

• Have gallstones or have family members with gallstones.

• Have obesity, high triglycerides (fat in the blood) or diabetes.

• Are a smoker.

• Are a heavy drinker (three or more drinks a day).

What causes pancreatitis?

Gallstones or heavy alcohol drinking are usually the cause of pancreatitis. Rarely, you can also get pancreatitis from:

- Medications (many can irritate the pancreas).

- High triglyceride levels (fat in the blood).

- Infections.

- Abdominal injury.

- Metabolic disorders such as diabetes.

- Genetic disorders such as cystic fibrosis.

What are the symptoms of pancreatitis?

Pancreatitis symptoms vary, depending on the type of condition:

Acute pancreatitis symptoms

If you have acute pancreatitis, you may experience:

- Moderate to severe upper abdominal pain that may spread to your back.

- Pain that comes on suddenly or builds up over a few days.

- Pain that worsens when eating.

- Swollen, tender abdomen.

- Nausea and vomiting.

- Fever.

- Faster than usual heart rate.

Chronic pancreatitis symptoms

Chronic pancreatitis may cause some of the same symptoms as acute pancreatitis. You may also develop:

- Constant, sometimes disabling pain that spreads to your back.

- Unexplained weight loss.

- Foamy diarrhea with visible oil droplets (steatorrhea).

- Diabetes (high blood sugar), if insulin-producing pancreas cells are damaged.

DIAGNOSIS AND TESTS

How is pancreatitis diagnosed?

Your provider may suspect pancreatitis based on your symptoms or risk factors, such as heavy alcohol use or gallstone disease. To confirm diagnosis, you may go through additional tests.

Diagnosing acute pancreatitis

For acute pancreatitis, your provider may order a blood test that measures the levels of two digestive enzymes (amylase and lipase) produced by the pancreas. High levels of these enzymes indicate acute pancreatitis. An ultrasound or computed tomography (CT scan) provides images of your pancreas, gall bladder and bile duct that can show abnormalities.

Diagnosing chronic pancreatitis

Diagnosing chronic pancreatitis is more involved. You may also need:

• Secretin pancreatic function test: This test checks for your pancreas's response to a hormone (secretin) released by the small intestine. Secretin usually triggers the pancreas to release a digestive juice. A medical professional passes a tube from your throat, through your stomach, into the upper part of the small intestine to insert secretin and measure the response.

• Oral glucose tolerance test: You may need this test if your provider suspects that pancreatitis has damaged your insulin-producing pancreas cells. It measures how your body handles sugar with a blood test before and after you drink a sugary liquid.

• Stool test: Your provider may order a stool test using a sample of your stool to see if your body is having difficulty breaking down fat.

• Endoscopic ultrasound (endosonography): An internal (endoscopic) ultrasound takes clearer pictures of your pancreas and connecting ducts (tubes). A healthcare professional inserts a thin tube with a tiny ultrasound attachment into your throat, through your stomach and into your small intestine. The endoscopic ultrasound takes detailed pictures of your internal organs including pancreas, part of liver, gall bladder and bile duct.

• ERCP (endoscopic retrograde cholangiopancreatography): A tube with a tiny camera is passed from your throat to your stomach and into your small intestine up to the area called the ampulla, where the pancreas and bile duct opens. Dye is injected into the pancreas duct and /or bile duct. The test lets your provider see inside the pancreas and bile duct. Anything blocking the pancreas or bile duct, such as a gallstone or pancreas stone, may be removed.

MANAGEMENT AND TREATMENT

How is pancreatitis treated?

If you have pancreatitis, your primary care provider will probably refer you to a specialist. A doctor who specializes in the digestive system (gastroenterologist) should oversee your care.

Doctors use one or more of these methods to treat acute pancreatitis:

• Hospitalization with supportive care and monitoring.

• Pain medication to provide comfort.

• Endoscopic procedure or surgery to remove a gallstone, other blockage or damaged part of the pancreas.

• Supplemental pancreatic enzymes and insulin, if your pancreas isn't functioning well.

Procedures used to treat pancreatitis

Most pancreatitis complications like pancreatic pseudocyst (type of inflammatory cyst) or infected pancreas tissue are managed through endoscopic procedure (inserting a tube down your throat until it reaches your small intestine, which is next to your pancreas). Gallstones and pancreas stones are removed with an endoscopic procedure.

If surgery is recommended, surgeons can often perform a laparoscopic procedure. This surgical technique involves smaller cuts that take less time to heal.

During laparoscopic surgery, your surgeon inserts a laparoscope (an instrument with a tiny camera and light) into keyhole-sized cuts in your abdomen. The laparoscope sends images of your organs to a monitor to help guide the surgeon during the procedure.

PREVENTION

Can pancreatitis be prevented?

The best way to prevent pancreatitis is to have a healthy lifestyle. Aim to:

- Maintain a healthy weight.

- Get regular exercise.

- Stop smoking.

- Avoid alcohol.

These healthy lifestyle choices will also help you avoid gallstones, which cause 40% of acute pancreatitis cases. Your provider may recommend removing your gallbladder if you have painful gallstones multiple times.

OUTLOOK / PROGNOSIS

How long does pancreatitis last?

Typically, acute pancreatitis lasts only a few days. But if you have a more severe case, it may take several weeks to months to recover. Chronic pancreatitis requires lifelong management.

Will pancreatitis go away?

With treatment, most people with acute pancreatitis completely recover.

Chronic pancreatitis is a long-lasting condition. Once it's severely damaged, your pancreas doesn't function properly. You need ongoing support to digest food and manage blood sugar.

Can pancreatitis return?

With chronic pancreatitis, painful episodes can come and go or persist (last a long time).

You can also have another attack of acute pancreatitis, especially if you haven't resolved the underlying problem. For example, if you have another gallstone that blocks the opening to the pancreas, you can get acute pancreatitis again.

Is pancreatitis fatal?

Most people with a mild case of acute pancreatitis fully recover. However, those with severe pancreatitis are more likely to have life-threatening complications such as:

• Infection of the pancreas.

• Bleeding in the pseudocyst or damaged pancreas.

• Heart, lung or kidney failure from spreading infection or if the pancreas leaks toxins into the blood.

LIVING WITH

How should I take care of myself after having pancreatitis?

You can take several steps to prevent another pancreatitis attack:

- Eat a low-fat diet.

- Stop drinking alcoholic beverages.

- Quit smoking.

- Follow your doctor's and nutritionist's dietary recommendations.

- Take medications as prescribed.

What should I ask my doctor?

If you have pancreatitis, you may want to ask your doctor:

- Do I have gallstones?

- Is my pancreas damaged?

- Are there any complications?

- Am I still producing insulin?

- What foods should I eat?

- What supplements should I take?

Pancreatitis Diet

Pancreatitis is an inflammation (swelling) of the pancreas. When the pancreas is inflamed, the powerful digestive enzymes it makes can damage its tissue. The inflamed pancreas can cause release of inflammatory cells and toxins that may harm your lungs, kidneys and heart.

Besides making insulin, which your body uses to regulate blood sugar, a healthy pancreas produces enzymes that help your body digest and make use of the food you eat. If your pancreas becomes inflamed (pancreatitis), it has a harder time breaking down fat and isn't able to absorb as much nutrition.

A pancreatitis diet takes this into account, prohibiting fatty foods and emphasizing choices that are nutrient-rich, especially those high in protein.

Changing how you eat, either temporarily or committing to a long-term pancreatitis diet, can help you manage your symptoms and prevent attacks, as well as keep you properly nourished despite your condition.

About 15% of people who have an episode of acute pancreatitis will have another. Chronic pancreatitis happens in closer to 5% of people.

Benefits

The most common cause of chronic pancreatitis is alcohol abuse, accounting for approximately 80% of cases.

Although diet does not directly cause pancreatitis (it can contribute to gallstones and increase lipid levels, both of which can lead to the condition, however), it can help treat symptoms and prevent future attacks in those who are diagnosed with the condition.

And the benefits go beyond comfort. A pancreatitis diet helps support an organ that's already functioning inefficiently, which is of great significance because a pancreas that becomes unable to contribute to insulin regulation can give way to developing diabetes.

Central to all of this is fat restriction. The less you consume, the less burden you put on your pancreas which, due to pancreatitis, is already challenged when it comes to metabolizing fat.

A 2013 study published in the journal Clinical Nutrition found that male patients with pancreatitis who ate a high-fat diet were more likely to have ongoing abdominal pain. They were also more likely to be diagnosed with chronic pancreatitis at a younger age.

Furthermore, a 2015 review of treatment guidelines developed by researchers in Japan found that patients with severe chronic pancreatitis benefitted from a very low-fat diet, but people with milder cases usually tolerated dietary fat (especially if they took digestive enzymes with meals).

If you have recurrent attacks of pancreatitis and continued pain, your doctor may have you experiment with your daily fat intake to see if your symptoms improve.

The pancreatitis diet's promotion of nutrient-dense foods also helps you thwart the possibility of malnourishment. One reason this can happen is that several key vitamins (A, D, and E) are fat-soluble; issues with fat digestion beget issues with properly absorbing these nutrients.

Being deficient in one or more fat-soluble vitamins comes with its own set of symptoms and health risks. For example, vitamin A deficiency can cause night blindness and vitamin

D deficiency has been linked to an increased risk of osteoporosis (especially after menopause).

How It Works

While the specifics of a pancreatitis diet plan will depend on your dietary needs and preferences, there are some general guidelines you can use as a starting point.

It's generally recommended that you avoid choices that are:

- High in fat

- Heavily processed

- Have a lot of sugar

- Contain alcohol

The guidelines for fat intake if you have pancreatitis vary. For example, the Digestive Health Center at Stanford University recommends patients with chronic pancreatitis limit fat intake to 30 to 50 grams per day, depending on how well it's tolerated.

Fat is still an important part of a balanced diet—you just may need to start paying more attention to and adjusting your intake of the kind of fat you eat.

For example, a type of fat called medium-chain triglycerides (MCTs) can be digested without any help from your pancreas. Coconut and coconut oil are naturally rich sources of MCTs, but it's also available in supplement form.

If your body is struggling to process healthy fats, your doctor might suggest you take digestive enzymes. These synthetic enzymes help make up for what your pancreas can't produce. They usually come in a capsule that you take when you eat.

Approaches

There are two overall approaches to managing pancreatitis with your diet. You may find you need to use both, depending on whether you are having an attack of symptoms or trying to prevent inflammation.

- When you're having acute pancreatitis symptoms, eating a limited diet of easily digested foods can be soothing.

• If you are in the middle of an acute attack, your doctor may want you to be on a limited diet of soft foods until your body heals.

For most mild cases of pancreatitis, complete bowel rest or a liquid-only diet is not necessary. A 2016 review of clinical guidelines for treating acute pancreatitis found that a soft diet was safe for most patients who were unable to tolerate their typical diet due to pancreatitis symptoms.

When symptoms of pancreatitis are severe or there are complications, a feeding tube or other methods of artificial nutrition may be necessary.

Duration

While you may be able to return to a less restricted diet once you are feeling better, doing so can cause symptoms to return. If you tend to have recurrent bouts of pancreatitis, changing how you eat for the long-term can help prevent attacks while ensuring you're probably nourished and hydrated.

What to Eat

Compliant

- Air-popped popcorn (without butter/oil), wheat or spelt pretzels

- Beans, lentils, legumes

- Coconut/palm kernel oil (for MCTs)

- Corn or whole-wheat tortillas

- Couscous, quinoa, whole wheat pasta

- Dairy-free milk alternatives (almond, soy, rice)

- Egg whites

- Fish (cod, haddock)

- Fresh/frozen/canned fruits and vegetables

- Fruit and vegetable juice without sugar or carbonation

- Herbal tea, decaffeinated coffee (with small amounts of honey or non-dairy creamer, if desired)

- Lean cuts of meat

- Low-fat or non-fat dairy products (cottage cheese, Greek yogurt)

- Low-fat sweets (graham crackers, ginger snaps, tea biscuits)

- Nutritional supplement drinks (Boost, Ensure)

- Poultry (turkey, chicken) without the skin

- Reduced sugar jams and jellies

- Rice

- Low-fat/fat-free clear soups and broth (avoid milk-based or creamy types)

- Spices and fresh herbs (as tolerated), salsa, tomato-based sauces

- Steel-cut oats, bran, farina, grits

- Sugar-free gelatin, ice pops

- Tofu, tempeh

- Tuna (canned in water not oil)

- Whole grain bread, cereals, and crackers

Non-Compliant

- Alcohol

- Baked goods (doughnuts, muffins, bagels, biscuits, croissants)

- Battered/fried fish and shellfish

- Butter, lard, vegetable oil, margarine, ghee

- Cake, pies, pastries

- Cheese, cream cheese, cheese sauce

- Cookies, brownies, candy

- Eggs with yolk

- Fatty cuts of red meat, organ meat

- Fried foods/fast food (stir-fried vegetables, fried rice, fried eggs, French fries)

- Ice cream, pudding, custards, milkshakes, smoothies with dairy

- Jams, jellies, preserves

- Lamb, goose, duck

- Milk-based coffee drinks

- Nut butters (peanut, almond)

- Nuts and seeds (in moderation as tolerated)

- Potato or corn chips

- Processed meat (sausage, hot dogs, lunchmeat)

- Refined white flour options (e.g., bread, pancakes, waffles, granola, cereal, crackers, pretzels)

- Refried beans, olives

- Store-bought salad dressing, mayo, creamy pasta sauces (Alfredo), tahini

- Whole milk, full-fat dairy products

• Soda, energy drinks

Fruits and vegetables: Choose produce with plenty of fiber, whether fresh or frozen. Canned fruits and vegetables can also work well, though you'll want to drain and rinse them to reduce the sugar/salt content. High-fat produce like avocados may be too rich for you to digest if you have pancreatitis.

Dairy: Choose low-fat or fat-free milk and yogurt or dairy-free alternatives such as almond, soy, and rice milk. Most types of cheese are high in fat, though lower-fat options like cottage cheese may not worsen your symptoms and can be a good source of protein.

Protein: Look for low-fat sources of protein to include in your pancreatitis diet such as white fish and lean cuts of skinless poultry. Beans, legumes, and lentils, as well as grains like quinoa, also make easy and tasty protein-packed meals. Nuts and nut butters are rich plant-based protein sources, but the high fat content may contribute to pancreatitis symptoms.

Grains: For the most part, you'll want to build your pancreatitis diet around fiber-rich whole grains. The exception can be when you're having symptoms and your doctor advises you to eat a bland diet, during which time you may find white rice, plain noodles, and white bread toast are easier to digest.

Desserts: Rich sweets, especially those made from milk like ice cream and custards, are usually too rich for people with pancreatitis.

Avoid high-sugar desserts like cakes, cookies, pastries, baked goods, and candy.

Depending on how well your body can regulate blood sugar, it may be fine to add honey or a little sugar to tea or black coffee, or to occasionally eat a small piece of dark chocolate.

Beverages: Alcohol must be completely avoided. If caffeinated tea, coffee, and soft drinks contribute to symptoms, you may choose to limit or avoid them as well. In general, avoiding soda will help you cut back on sugar in your diet. If you continue to drink coffee, avoid milk-based drinks with sweetened syrups.

Hydration is important and, as always, water is the best choice. Herbal tea, fruit and vegetable juices, and nutritional supplement drinks recommended by your doctor are a few other options.

Recommended Timing

If you have pancreatitis, you may find that you feel better adhering to a certain eating schedule. Try eating several small meals and snacks throughout the day instead of three large ones.

If you tend to feel full quickly, it can also be helpful to avoid eating and drinking at the same time. You may also feel better if you avoid combining certain foods or ingredients; take note of how you feel after meals and make adjustments as needed.

Cooking Tips

Avoid fried, sautéed, or stir-fried foods. Instead, try baking, grilling, roasting, boiling, and steaming. Fats like butter, lard, and oils are best avoided, though you may tolerate small amounts for cooking.

Certain spices may be irritating, but turmeric and ginger are tasty and have digestive benefits.

Considerations

In some cases, people with pancreatitis try to prevent symptoms by restricting their diet on their own, which also contributes to malnutrition. While there are foods that can make pancreatitis worse, there are also plenty of nutritious foods that also promote digestive health and may help reduce inflammation.

For example, plant-based and lean sources of animal protein, whole grains, and fiber-rich produce provide key vitamins and minerals your body can use for energy without putting too much stress on your digestive system.

A nutritionist can help you make choices that manage your condition and keep you healthy. Maintaining adequate nutrition is especially important in cases of severe pancreatitis, as the body's energy needs may actually increase.

Research has shown that when patients with pancreatitis are underweight or critically ill from infections like sepsis, the amount of energy their bodies use at rest (resting energy expenditure) can increase by up to 50%.

Modifications and Dietary Restrictions

If you have other health conditions, you may need to adjust your pancreatitis diet to ensure you're getting the nutrition you need. It's important that you share any other diagnoses you have with your healthcare team and seek help devising a diet that both manages your pancreatitis and other issue(s).

For example, attacks of pancreatitis can occur during pregnancy. Your dietary needs will be different when you're pregnant or nursing, however, so your plan may need to be adjusted accordingly.

Nutrition is also an important consideration if you have another medical condition that affects your digestion. For example, if you have inflammatory bowel disease or cystic fibrosis, you may already have issues with malabsorption. Having gallbladder disease means you are more likely to have digestive symptoms.

If you also have diabetes, your pancreas is already working extra hard—or not working well at all. In this case, the decisions you make about what you eat and drink will have an even greater effect on your overall health.

Additionally, people who have high levels of triglycerides (hypertriglyceridemia) may have stricter parameters in terms of avoiding or limiting foods that are high in saturated fats.

Flexibility

If you're dining out and are not sure how much fat is in a particular dish you're considering, ask your server. You may be able to lower the fat content by asking for swaps or substitutions, or splitting a dish with someone.

Be sure to read labels when you shop at the grocery store. For the most part, you'll want to look for products that are low-fat and fat-free. These days, there are many, making the diet easier to follow. Remember, though: While nutrition labels list the amount of fat per serving, a package may contain more than one serving.

Support and Community

If you're feeling frustrated by or disappointed about the need to change how you eat, it can be helpful to talk to other people who have been through what you're experiencing.

Joining an in-person or online support group is one way to connect with other people managing pancreatitis through diet. What works for them may not work for you, but sharing ideas and support one another can help you keep up your motivation.

Cost

If your doctor wants you to take nutritional supplements, you'll find the price of vitamins varies considerably based on type, brand, and dose. If you develop exocrine pancreatic insufficiency and your doctor wants you to start pancreatic enzyme replacement therapy (PERT), this can be another added cost.

Much like nutritional and vitamin supplements, you may be able to find PERT capsules at most pharmacies and health food stores. The product you'll need to purchase will depend on the combination of enzymes and amount (units) your doctor wants you to take with each meal.

If you have health insurance, ask your doctor if they can prescribe vitamins, nutritional supplements, or PERT. Your insurance may cover part or all of the cost. However, with PERT, coverage may be limited based on FDA approval.

One-day sample pancreatitis diet

Here is a one-day sample pancreatitis diet that contains plenty of fruits and vegetables, lean proteins, and whole-grains.

This sample diet also contains smaller, more frequent snacks and meals to help promote better digestion and reduce stomach discomfort.

Breakfast

- 1 cup (80 grams) of oatmeal cooked with water

- banana, sliced for oatmeal topping

- 1 whole egg and three egg whites with diced peppers

Snack

- 1 cup (227 grams) of low-fat cottage cheese

- 1 cup (140 grams) of blueberries

Lunch

- a sandwich made with:

- 3 ounces (85 grams) of lean deli turkey breast

- 1 slice of low-fat Swiss cheese

- mustard

- tomato slice

- shredded lettuce

- apple slices

Snack

- herbed yogurt dip made with:

- 1 cup (227 grams) plain Greek yogurt

- green onion, minced

- parsley, finely chopped

- fresh dill, chopped

- fresh chives, chopped

- basil, thinly sliced

- lemon juice

- fresh vegetables for dipping

Dinner

- a fish taco made with:

- 4 ounces (113 grams) of tilapia, baked and shredded

- avocado, sliced

- tomato, sliced

- red onion, diced

- purple cabbage, sliced

- sour cream

- mayo

- lime juice

- salt and pepper to taste

PANCREATITIS DIET RECIPES

In this part are pancreatitis diet recipes to help keep your pancreatitis at bay

APPLE BUTTERNUT SQUASH PANCAKES

Preparation time

15 minutes

INGREDIENTS:

• 3 cups grated raw butternut squash or acorn squash (may also use zucchini)

• 1 large green apple (or 2 small) grated, raw

- 1/3 cup sour cream (use reduced-fat or vegan sour cream if necessary)

- 1 egg

- 1/4 cup milk of choice (use lactose-free, non-dairy, or reduced-fat as needed)

- 1 cup all-purpose flour

- 1 tsp. baking powder

- 1 tsp. baking soda

- 1 tsp. cinnamon

Instructions

1. Grate squash on cheese grater or food processor.

2. Steam in a shallow bowl in microwave with a small amount of water for 3 minutes to soften.

3. Core and grate apple on cheese grater or food processor, and add to squash mixture.

4. Add squash and apple to a mixing bowl and stir in sour cream, egg, and milk with a fork.

5. In a separate bowl, sift flour, baking powder, baking soda, and cinnamon.

6. Add to mixing bowl and stir with the fork.

7. Heat frying pan to low-medium and spray with cooking spray.

8. Using a ladle or a spoon, drop batter onto pan into small pancakes.

9. Flip when bubbles start to form around the edges of pancake.

CARROT AND SWEET POTATO SOUP

WITH CRANBERRY RELISH

Preparation time

1 hour

Ingredients

RELISH:

- 1/4 cup fresh cranberries, coarsely chopped

- 3 tablespoons fresh orange juice

- 1 tablespoon chopped shallots (1 medium)

- 1/2 teaspoon sugar

SOUP:

- 2 large carrots, peeled and cut in 2-inch pieces (about 4 1/2 ounces)

- 1 large sweet potato, peeled and cut in 2-inch chunks (about 3/4 pound)

- 1 small onion, cut into 8 wedges (about 14 ounces)

- 1 tablespoon olive oil

- 4 cups organic vegetable broth (such as Swanson Certified Organic)

- 1 teaspoon finely grated fresh ginger

- 1/4 teaspoon salt

- 1/4 teaspoon freshly ground black pepper

REMAINING INGREDIENT:

• 2 tablespoons chopped fresh flat-leaf parsley

Instructions

1. To prepare relish, combine the first 4 ingredients in a small bowl; set aside.

2. Preheat oven to 400°.

3. To prepare soup, combine carrots, sweet potato, and onion on a jelly-roll pan; drizzle with oil.

4. Toss to coat.

5.   Bake at 400° for 30 minutes or until vegetables are tender and just beginning to brown, stirring after 15 minutes.

6. Place vegetables, broth, and ginger in a Dutch oven over medium-high heat; bring to a boil.

7. Cover, reduce heat, and simmer for 20 minutes.

8. Place half of vegetable mixture in a blender.

9. Remove center piece of blender lid (to allow steam to escape); secure blender lid on blender.

10. Place a clean towel over opening in blender lid (to avoid splatters).

11. Blend until smooth.

12.   Pour pureed mixture into a large bowl; repeat procedure with remaining vegetable mixture.

13. Stir in salt and pepper.

14. Ladle 1 cup soup into each of 4 bowls. Stir parsley into relish. Top each serving with 1 tablespoon relish mixture.

LIME-SPIKED BLACK BEAN DIP

Preparation time

INGREDIENTS

- 2 (15-ounce) cans black beans, rinsed and drained

- 1 cup grated carrot

- 1/2 cup fresh lime juice (about 2 limes)

- 1/4 cup finely chopped green onions

- 1/4 cup chopped fresh cilantro

- 1 teaspoon minced garlic

- 1/4 teaspoon salt

- 1/8 teaspoon ground red pepper

INSTRUCTIONS

1. Place beans in a food processor, and pulse until almost smooth. Combine the beans, carrot, and the remaining ingredients in a medium bowl,

stirring until well blended. Let stand 30 minutes.

Serve with baked tortilla chips.

LENTIL STEW

Preparation time

1 hour

Ingredients

- 1 small onion, chopped

- 2-3 Tbs. Olive oil

- (Optional: add one clove garlic, minced)

- 8 cups vegetable broth

- 1 cup lentils

- 2 bay leaves

- ½ cup basmati rice

- 2 medium carrots, chopped

- 1 small yam or sweet potato, peeled and chopped

- 1 bunch spinach or Swiss chard

- 1 grated zucchini

- 1 small bunch basil, chopped

- 2 tsp. ground cumin

- 1 tsp. ground coriander

- ½ tsp. cinnamon

- Salt, to taste

Instructions

1. Sauté onion in olive oil until slightly golden brown. (Optional: Add one clove garlic,

2. minced.)

3. Add vegetable broth, lentils, and bay leaves.

4. Bring to a boil, then lower heat and simmerfor 20 minutes.

5. Add rice, carrots, and sweet potato.

6. Simmer 15 minutes.

7. Add water if the stew looks too thick.

8. Add spinach, zucchini, basil, cumin, coriander, cinnamon, and salt to taste. Simmer until all ingredients are tender, 10 to 15 minutes. Serve

CITRUS CHICKEN WITH OREGANO AND CUMIN

Preparation time

40 minutes

Ingredients:

- 4 boneless chicken breast

- 1 tablespoon dried oregano

- 1 teaspoon ground cumin

- 2 garlic cloves, minced

- zest and juice of 1 lime

- zest and juice of 1 orange

- 1 teaspoon of kosher salt

- 1/2 teaspoon black pepper

- 1 tablespoon vegetable or olive oil

Instructions

1. Place the chicken, oregano, cumin, garlic, and zest and juice of lime and orange in a large non-reactive shallow bowl and stir to combine.

2. Cover and refrigerate at least 1/2 hour and not more than one hour.

3. Remove and discard as much of the marinade as possible.

4. Sprinkle the chicken with salt and pepper.

5. Place a large cast iron or non stick skillet over high heat and when it is hot, add the oil.

6. Add the chicken breasts one at a time, waiting about 30 seconds between additions.

7. Cook until well browned and cooked throughout.

8. Transfer the chicken to a platter and serve immediately.

Tangy Skillet Chicken

Preparation time

30 minutes

INGREDIENTS

- 4 teaspoons extra-virgin olive oil

- 1 tablespoon fresh or bottled garlic, minced

- 3 tablespoons Meyer lemon juice (or substitute regular lemon juice)

- 4 tablespoons water, or chicken broth or white wine

- 4 boneless, skinless chicken breast halves, (unfold the tenderloin area to make the breast as flat as possible)

- freshly ground black pepper

INSTRUCTIONS

1. Add olive oil to a large, nonstick skillet and begin to heat over medium-high heat.

2. When hot (a minute or two), add garlic and chicken breasts (placing them so they are nice and flat and covering the olive oil in the bottom of the skillet). Brown for two-three minutes,

sprinkle the top with pepper, then flip to brown the other side for two to three minutes.

3. Turn heat down to low and drizzle the lemon juice and water, chicken broth, or wine over the top.

4. Cover skillet immediately and cook until chicken is cooked throughout (about 15 more minutes).

5. Serve the chicken with or without the lemon broth in the bottom of the skillet.

Chicken-A-La-King

Preparation time

55 minutes

Ingredients

- 4 large Chicken Fillets

- 2 cups Water

- 2 cubes Low-Salt Chicken Stock

- 1 Onion, chopped

- 1/2 Red Bell Pepper, chopped

- 1/2 Green Bell Pepper, chopped

- 250 g Mushrooms, sliced (8 oz)

- 1 cup Frozen Peas

- 1 packet White Onion Soup Powder

- 1 cup Fat-Free Milk

- 1/2 t Paprika

Instructions

1. Cook the Chicken in the Water and Stock cubes until fully cooked – remove the Chicken and cut into bite size pieces – retain 2/3 cup of the Chicken Stock

2. Fry the Onion, Peppers and Mushrooms in a non-stick pan until soft – add the Chicken, the retained Stock and the Peas – cover and simmer 5 minutes

3. Mix the Soup Powder, Milk and Paprika – add to the Chicken – cover and simmer over low heat for another 10 – 15 minutes

Tomato and Vegetable Red Lentil Soup

Preparation time

35 minutes

Ingredients

• 2 teaspoons olive oil

• 450g packet soup mix vegetables (eg onion, carrot, celery, swede, potato) cut into 1cm cubes

• 800g can diced tomatoes

- 3 cups liquid vegetable salt

- ½ cup red split lentils

- Salt and pepper

Instructions

1. In a large saucepan heat oil over a medium heat , add chopped vegetables and cook until slightly soft.

2. Add tomatoes, stock and lentils, bring to the boil then reduce heat and simmer for about 15-20 minutes until the lentils are tender.

3. Add a sprinkle of salt and pepper.

Tweaks

1. Add some finely chopped garlic and fresh coriander for extra flavour.

2. Serve with crusty bread for dunking.

Flourless Chocolate Cupcakes with Spiced Sweet Potato Frosting

Preparation time

50 minutes

Ingredients

- 1/2 cup millet 105

- 1/2 cup buckwheat groats 100g

- 1 apple cored and cut into eights

- 1/2 cup unsweetened dried coconut 25g

- 1/2 cup 100% pure maple syrup 120 ml

- 1/2 cup cacao powder 30g

- 3/4 cup mineral water 175 ml

- 1/2 cup walnuts 50

- 1 teaspoon baking powder

- 1/2 teaspoon baking soda

Frosting

- 1/2 cup cooked sweet potato 110g

- 1/4 cups walnuts 20g

- 3 dates pits taken out and simmered for at least 5 minutes in water

- 1/2 tablespoon 100% pure maple syrup

- 1/8 teaspoon cinnamon

Instructions

1. Soak the millet and the buckwheat overnight or for an entire day.

2. Preheat the oven to 350°F (175°C).

3. Drain and rinse the grains and add them to the blender along with the apple, coconut, maple syrup, cacao powder, mineral water, and walnuts.

4. Blend until totally smooth, about 3 minutes.

5. Pour the batter into a mixing bowl, add the baking powder and the baking soda, and whisk just until incorporated.

6. Line your muffin tin with liners and fill each one with batter.

7. Bake for 35 minutes.

8. While the cupcakes are baking, make the frosting.

9. Place the cooked sweet potato, walnuts, dates, maple syrup, and cinnamon into the blender and blend until totally creamy and smooth, about 2 minutes.

10. Put the frosting in the fridge until the cupcakes are out of the oven and totally cool.

11. When the cupcakes are cool, spread a generous amount of frosting on each.

Lentil Vegetable Soup with Turmeric

Preparation time

30 minutes

Ingredients

- 1/2 onion chopped

- 1 cup dried red lentils

- 2 carrots peeled and chopped

- 2 celery stalks chopped

- 2 tbsp parsley

- 3 cups spring water (+additional 1/2 cup for pureeing)

- 1 tsp turmeric

- 1/4 tsp Himalayan salt (or sea salt)

Instructions

1. Add all ingredients to the medium size pot and bring to a boil.

2. Cover and reduce the heat to low.

3. Simmer for 25 minutes.

FOR PUREED VERSION:

1. Cool the soup to room temperature in the refrigerator, then add to a blender in 2 batches.

2. Add additional 1/4 cup water to each batch before blending.

3. DO NOT PUT HOT LIQUID to your Magic Bullet! Blend for 10-15 seconds. Serve hot or cold.

Shredded Chicken Tacos

Preparation time

3 hours

Ingredients

- 1 (14.5 ounce) can fire-roasted diced tomatoes, undrained

- 1 fresh jalapeño pepper, halved and stemmed (see Tip)

- 3 cloves garlic, peeled

- 2 tablespoons chili powder

- 1 tablespoon ground cumin

- ½ teaspoon salt

- 2 pounds skinless, boneless chicken thighs

- 16 (6 inch) corn or flour tortillas, warmed

- 1 cup Guacamole, chopped fresh cilantro, and/or lime wedges

Instructions

1. Combine undrained tomatoes, jalapeño pepper, garlic, chili powder, and salt in a blender;

2. cover and blend until smooth.

3. Pour the tomato mixture into a 3 1/2- to 4-quart slow cooker.

4. Add chicken thighs; stir to coat.

5. Cover and cook on Low for 5 to 6 hours or on High for 2 1/2 to 3 hours.

6. Remove the chicken and place in a bowl.

7. Shred the chicken using two forks.

8. Add enough sauce mixture from the slow cooker to the shredded chicken to moisten.

9. Serve the chicken in tortillas.

10. If desired, top with guacamole, cilantro, and/or lime wedges.

Lentil Pasta Sauce

Preparation time

1 hour

INGREDIENTS

- 1 tablespoon extra virgin olive oil

- 1 medium onion, diced

- 3 garlic cloves, minced

- 1-28 ounce can crushed tomatoes

- 1-28 ounce can fire roasted tomatoes

- 1 tablespoon fresh parsley, chopped

- 1 tablespoon Italian seasoning

- 2 bay leaves

- 1 cup dry lentils

INSTRUCTIONS

1. Heat oil to medium high in a large sauce pan.

2. Saute onion and garlic until translucent about four minutes.

3. Add crushed tomatoes, fire roasted tomatoes, parsley, Italian seasoning, and bay leaves.

4. Bring to a boil and simmer for 30 minutes.

5. While sauce is cooking, add lentils to a medium sauce pan with 3 cups of water.

6. Bring to a boil, cover, and reduce the heat to a simmer.

7. Simmer for 15-20 minutes until lentils are tender and drain.

8. When sauce is finished cooking mix in cooked lentils and serve.

9. Enjoy over pasta, roast vegetables, or toast.

Healthy Lemon Garlic Salmon

Preparation time

15 minutes

INGREDIENTS

- 4 salmon portions skin-on

- 1/2 teaspoon salt

- 1/2 teaspoon black pepper

- 2 teaspoons extra virgin olive oil

- 4 tablespoons fresh lemon juice

- 8 garlic cloves crushed

- 2 tablespoons finely chopped fresh dill

INSTRUCTIONS

1. Season salmon portions with salt and pepper.

2. Heat a large heavy skillet over medium-high heat.

3. Add in olive oil and heat 30 seconds.

4. Place salmon portions into the skillet, starting with the skin side up.

5. Sear 3 to 4 minutes, then flip over and sear the other side 3 more minutes.

6. Move salmon to one side of the pan.

7. Pour lemon juice into empty area of skillet and in garlic cloves and saute 60 seconds.

8. Spoon garlic lemon juice over salmon and cook until fish is cooked through and flakes easily with a fork.

9. Sprinkle fresh dill on top of salmon portions and serve immediately.

10. Garnish with lemon slices if desired.

FavoritePeaches & Cream Smoothie

Preparation time

5 minutes

Ingredients

• 1/2 cup rolled oats

• 1/3 cup plain yogurt (or soy/coconut/almond yogurt)

• 3/4 cup milk (or soy/almond/rice milk) + 1/4 cup more for morning

- 1 small ripe peach (or 1/2 cup frozen peaches, thawed and softened)

- 1/2 medium banana

- 1-2 tbsp protein powder (whey or soy) (optional)

- Pinch of salt

Instructions

1. Gather all ingredients.

2. Combine ingredients in a blender and enjoy.

3. Store in a container in your refrigerator overnight if making ahead of time.

4. In the morning, add last 1/4 cup milk, more if you need it to blend smoothly.

Low Sugar Blueberry Smoothie

Preparation time

5 minutes

INGREDIENTS

- 1 cup fresh or frozen wild blueberries

- 1/2 banana

- 1 cup frozen cauliflower florets

- 1/4 avocado

- 1 cup water , plus more as needed

- 1 tablespoon lemon juice

INSTRUCTIONS

1. Combine all of the ingredients in a high speed blender and blend until smooth and creamy.

2. Add more water as needed, then serve immediately.

CHOCOLATE BANANA SMOOTHIE

Preparation time

5 minutes

INGREDIENTS

- 1 frozen banana (120 g)

- 2 tbsp raw cacao powder (12 g)

- 1 tbsp chia seeds (10 g)

- 1 tbsp ground flax (8 g)

- handful of greens such as spinach or kale (40 g)

- 1/2 tsp quality sea salt

- 1 serving vegan vanilla protein powder (30 g)

- 1 1/2 cups unsweetened almond milk

- 1 tsp gelatinized maca powder

- optional: 1 tsp mesquite powder

INSTRUCTIONS

1. Add all ingredients to a high-speed blender and blend on max for 30-60 seconds until completely smooth and creamy.

2. Pour into a glass and enjoy with a glass or stainless steel straw.

Banana Spice Smoothie

Preparation time

5 minutes

Ingredients

- 2 ripe bananas

- 2 cups vanilla kefir (see Tip)

- ½ teaspoon ground cinnamon

- ⅛ teaspoon ground nutmeg

- ⅛ teaspoon ground allspice

- 12 ice cubes

Instructions

1. Combine kefir, bananas, cinnamon, nutmeg, allspice and ice cubes in a blender;

2. blend until smooth.

3. Serve immediately.

summerberry smoothie

Preparation time

Ingredients

- 50g frozen raspberries

- 50g frozen strawberries

- 200ml skimmed milk

- sugar-free and calorie-free sweetener, to taste

Instructions

1. Place the berries and the milk in a food processor or blender

2. Blend until smooth and frothy

3. Sweeten to taste and serve.

Coconutty Fig Smoothie

Preparation time

5 minutes

Ingredients

- 1 cup cauliflower

- 2 large spoonfuls coconut butter

- 1 fresh fig

- 1 tablespoon flaxseeds

- 1 scoop vanilla protein powder

- dash cinnamon

- 1/3 cup milk your choice coconut milk would be best – she made coconut collagen milk

- topped with a few fig slices grain-free granola and coconut flakes

Instructions

1. Blend all ingredients together until smooth

Smoky Jalapeño Hibiscus Cooler

Preparation time

5 minutes

Ingredients

- Spice Glass Rim: (optional)

- 1/2 lime

- 1 tsp. sugar

- 1/4 tsp. cinnamon

- 1/4 tsp. smoked paprika

Cooler:

- 1/2 cup orange juice, unsweetened

- 1 small lime, juiced

- 1/4-1/2 small jalapeño, sliced (depending on heat preference)

- 1/2 tsp. smoked paprika

- 1 12-ounce can hibiscus flavored sparkling water, unsweetened*

- 1 large or 6 small ice cubes

Garnish: (optional)

- Orange, lime slices

- Jalapeño slices

- Hibiscus flowers

Instructions

1. Create a spice glass rim with two 12-ounce glasses by running lime halfway along edge of each glass.

2. Mix sugar, cinnamon and paprika together in small saucer.

3. Press each glass into spice mixture to coat rims.

4. Allow to dry for a few minutes before adding liquid to glasses.

5. Or use plain glasses.

6. Place orange juice, lime juice, jalapeño and smoked paprika in blender. Process for 1-2 minutes until well blended.

7. Place ice cubes in each glass.

8. Divide blended juice mixture between each glass.

9. Top each glass with half of hibiscus flavored sparkling water.

10. Garnish with orange, lime and jalapeño slices and hibiscus flowers, if desired.

Peanut Butter Toast with Banana and Chia Seeds

Preparation time

5 minutes

Ingredients

- 1 slice whole grain bread

- 1 Tbsp. peanut butter

- 1/2 banana, sliced

- 1 tsp. chia seed (or flaxseed)

Instructions

1. Toast bread.

2. Spread peanut butter on toast.

3. Top with sliced banana and chia seeds.

Peanut Butter Banana "Ice Cream"

Preparation time

2 hours

Ingredients

• 4 large ripe bananas, sliced

• 2 Tbsp. peanut butter (or other nut butter, such as almond butter)

• 1/4 tsp. vanilla extract

• 1/4 tsp. salt

- 1/2 tsp. cinnamon

- 2 Tbsp. chopped peanuts, for topping

Instructions

1. Slice bananas into chunks and freeze on a flat sheet pan (with pieces separated so they don't stick together) until solid, for at least 1-2 hours.

2. Add the frozen bananas to blender or food processor and blend until smooth and creamy.

3. This will take a few minutes with periodic pauses to stir/scrape down bananas in blender/food processor.

4. Once bananas have reached a creamy texture, add peanut butter, vanilla extract, salt and cinnamon and continue to blend.

5. Scoop into individual bowls and top with chopped peanuts.

6. Serve immediately.

Oatmeal with Fresh Fruit

Preparation time

15 minutes

Ingredients

- 1/2 cup old fashioned rolled oats

- 1 1/4 cups almond milk, divided*

- 1 tsp. ground flaxseed, or to taste

- 1/8 tsp. cinnamon

- 1/2 cup chopped pineapple

- 1/4 cup sliced strawberries

- 2 Tbsp. chopped walnuts, optional

- 1 tsp. honey, optional

Instructions

1. In small pan, cook oatmeal with 1 cup milk according to package directions.

2. Place oatmeal in serving bowl.

3. Pour ¼ cup milk over oatmeal (heat milk if preferred).

4. Sprinkle on flaxseed and cinnamon.

5. Top with pineapple, strawberries, walnuts and honey, if desired.

Polenta with Fruit Compote

Preparation time

20 minutes

Ingredients

- 3 cups warm water

- 1 cup cornmeal

- 1 cup cold water

- 3 Tbsp. maple syrup, divided

- 1/2 tsp. salt

- 3 cups frozen berries

Instructions

1. Add warm water to saucepan and bring to a boil over medium heat.

2. Meanwhile, mix cornmeal and cold water, stirring until combined.

3. To boiling water, add cornmeal mixture, 1 Tbsp. maple syrup and salt.

4. Reduce heat to simmer, cover and stir occasionally.

5. Cook for 10 minutes or until water is absorbed.

6. While cornmeal is simmering, add fruit and remaining 2 Tbsp. maple syrup to saucepan.

7. Heat over medium heat, until fruit cooks down into compote.

8. To serve, top cornmeal with fruit compote.

Apple Cinnamon Fruit Leather

Preparation time

3 hours 10 minutes

Ingredients

- 5 medium apples, chopped

- 1/2 cup water

- 1 large date, pitted

- 1 tsp cinnamon

Instructions

1. Place chopped apples in a medium saucepan with water.

2. Bring to a simmer, cover and cook for about 10 minutes.

3. Add pitted date and cinnamon and mash.

4. Cover and cook another 2-3 minutes on low heat.

5. Place mixture in a blender or food processor and process until smooth.

6. Pour onto a baking sheet lined with parchment paper or a non-stick baking mat and spread with a spatula into a thin layer.

7. Bake at 175-200° (as low as your oven will go) for 2-3 hours or until it's tacky but doesn't stick to your finger.

Fresh Cherry and Corn Salad

Preparation time

15 minutes

Ingredients

Dressing:

- 1/2 medium shallot, finely chopped

- 3 cloves garlic, minced

- 1/4 cup extra virgin olive oil

- 1/4 cup balsamic vinegar

- Salt and freshly ground black or white pepper to taste

Salad:

- 5 ounces baby arugula or baby spinach

- 4 ears cooked fresh corn, kernels sliced off cob

- 1/2 cup finely sliced red onion

- 3/4 cup feta cheese

- 1 lb fresh dark cherries, pitted, sliced in half

Instructions

1. In small mixing bowl, combine all dressing ingredients. Whisk well.

2. In large salad bowl combine arugula, corn and onion. Drizzle with dressing and toss to coat.

3. Arrange salad on individual dishes and sprinkle with feta. Top with cherries and serve.

Peach and Basil Salad with Fresh Mozzarella

Preparation time

10 minutes

Ingredients

- 1 lb. peaches, sliced into wedges, then cut crosswise (frozen may be used)

- 8 oz. part skimmed, fresh mozzarella cheese, cut into 3/4-inch cubes

- 1 cup loosely packed fresh basil, torn into medium pieces

- 2 tsp. extra virgin olive oil

- 2 tsp. rice vinegar

- Pinch salt

- Freshly ground black pepper, optional

Instructions

1. In large mixing bowl combine peaches, mozzarella and basil.

2. Drizzle on oil and vinegar, add salt and pepper, if using, and toss gently until evenly coated.

3. Serve immediately or refrigerate up to 4 hours.

Fresh and Light Veggie Pad Thai

Preparation time

45 minutes

Ingredients

Pad Thai

- 8 ounces dried wide, flat rice noodles (preferably brown rice noodles)

- 1 Tbsp. olive, sesame, or canola oil (divided)

- 8 ounces extra firm tofu, drained and cut into ½ inch cubes

- 2 large eggs

- 1/2 yellow onion, chopped

- 3 cloves garlic, minced

- 1 head of broccoli, cut into small florets

- 1 zucchini, spiralized (or sliced into thin, long strips)

- 1 cup snap peas

- 2 carrots, grated

- 1 cup mung bean sprouts

- 1/4 cup fresh basil, chopped

- 1/4 cup fresh cilantro, chopped

- Crushed red pepper, to taste

Sauce

- 1 Tbsp. fish sauce

- 2 Tbsp. rice vinegar

- 1 Tbsp. reduced sodium soy sauce or tamari (gluten-free)

- 1 Tbsp. honey (or sub another sweetener)

- 1/4 cup lime juice (juice of 1-2 limes)

Garnishes

- 2 Tbsp. peanuts, chopped

- Lime wedges

Instructions

1. Prepare the sauce by whisking together all the sauce ingredients in a small bowl and set aside.

2. Next, prepare the noodles according to package instructions.

3. For most rice noodles: bring a pot of water to a boil, remove from heat and let the noodles

soak in the hot water until just al dente (about 10 minutes).

4. Drain and set noodles aside.

5. Heat 1/2 of the oil over medium-high heat.

6. Sauté tofu about 3 minutes, or until just getting golden brown.

7. Rotate the pieces to get a golden color on all sides.

8. Move it to the edge of the pan.

9. Crack eggs into the pan, sauté with spatula to break yolk and scramble until just cooked through (about 1 min).

10. Set the egg and tofu aside on a plate for a later step.

11. Add the remaining oil to the pan and add the onion and garlic.

12. Sauté 1-2 minutes, or until just translucent.

13. Optional: add a pinch of red chili flakes for extra heat.

14. Sauté the rest of your vegetables until they are just fork-tender and still bright in color, about 3 minutes.

15. Add the noodles, sauce, and tofu/egg mixture to the pan.

16. Gently mix everything together so the flavors combine and the noodles can soak up the sauce.

17. Add most of the herbs and bean sprouts (reserve a handful for garnish).

18. Serve with a topping of fresh herbs, the remaining bean sprouts, lime wedges, and a sprinkle of peanuts.

Fresh Tomato Sauce

Preparation time

45 minutes

Ingredients

- 3 Ib ripe plum tomatoes

- 1 Tbsp. extra-virgin olive oil

- 3/4 cup finely chopped onion

- 1 large garlic clove, finely chopped

- 1 Tbsp. chopped fresh oregano, or 1 tsp. dried

- 1/2 tsp. sugar, optional

- 1 Tbsp. chopped fresh basil, or 1 tsp. dried

- Salt and freshly ground pepper, to taste

Instructions

1. Cut thin slice off top of tomatoes.

2. Peel tomatoes, using either serrated swivel-blade vegetable peeler or hot water method.*

3. Chop tomatoes and set aside; there will be 6-7 cups.

4. In large heavy pot, heat oil over medium-high heat.

5. Add onion and cook for 3 minutes, stirring occasionally.

6. Add garlic and cook, stirring often, until onion starts to color, 3-4 minutes.

7. Add tomatoes and oregano and stir well.

8. Cook, uncovered, for 15 minutes.

9. Taste sauce, adding sugar if it is too acidic.

10. Mix in basil and cook until tomatoes have broken down to your taste, 10-15 minutes for chunky sauce, 12-15 minutes for pulpier sauce.

11. Add salt and pepper, to taste.

Strawberry Aguas Frescas

Preparation time

10 minutes

Ingredients

- 2 cups sliced fresh strawberries

- 2 cups water

- 2 limes, juiced

- 1 tsp. agave nectar (optional)

- Ice cubes

- Garnish (optional)

- Additional strawberries

- Fresh mint leaves

Instructions

1. Place strawberries, water, lime juice and agave nectar (if using) in the container of a blender.

2. Process a few seconds until smooth.

3. Fill 2 large glasses or a small pitcher with ice cubes.

4. Pour aguas frescas into glasses or the entire batch into pitcher.

5. Garnish with fresh, whole strawberries and mint leaves, if desired.

Oatmeal Chocolate Chip Bites

Preparation time

25 minutes

Ingredients

• 2 cups old fashioned oats

- 1 cup almond flour

- 3/4 cup ground flaxseed

- 1/2 tsp. salt

- 2 tsp. baking powder

- 1/2 cup mini unsweetened chocolate chips

- 2 tsp. vanilla extract

- 1 cup pure maple syrup

- 1/2 cup natural almond butter

Instructions

1. Preheat oven to 350 degrees F.

2. Combine dry ingredients including chocolate chips in large bowl.

3. In another bowl, mix wet ingredients.

4. Add wet ingredients to dry ingredients and stir to combine.

5. Drop dough into 24 even mounds on greased baking sheet.

6. Lightly press down to flatten (cookies will not flatten much during cooking).

7. Or pour batter into greased 9 x 13-inch baking pan.

8. Bake 12-15 minute, until cookies are set in the center.

Anzac Cookies

Preparation time

2 hours 40 minutes

Ingredients

- 1 cup quick-cooking rolled oats

- 1 cup reduced-fat, unsweetened shredded dried coconut

- 1/2 cup whole-wheat pastry flour

- 1/2 cup unbleached all-purpose flour

- 1/2 cup granulated sugar

- 1/4 cup packed brown sugar

- 1/2 tsp. salt

- 1/2 cup buttery spread

- 2 Tbsp. honey

- 1/2 tsp. baking soda

- 2 Tbsp. boiling water

- Canola oil cooking spray

Instructions

1. In mixing bowl, use whisk to combine oats, coconut, flours, sugars and salt.

2. In small pot over medium heat, heat buttery spread until melted.

3. Mix in honey.

4. Remove pot from heat.

5. In small bowl, combine baking soda with boiling water.

6. When mixture is foamy, add to melted spread mixture.

7. Pour warm mixture into dry ingredients and mix, first using flexible spatula, then your hands, working with your fingers until mixture is evenly moistened.

8. It will be sandy and crumble when squeezed in your fist.

9. Cover bowl with plastic wrap and set aside at room temperature for 2-24 hours, until handful squeezed tightly sticks together.

10. Preheat oven to 325 degrees.

11. Coat 11-inch x 7-inch baking pan with cooking spray.

12. Pour bar mixture into prepared pan and press firmly into even layer.

13. Bake 10 minutes.

14. Remove pan and using sharp, thin knife make 4 cuts spaced evenly across wider width of pan.

15. Rotate pan 90 degrees and make 3 cuts across smaller width of pan, creating 20 bars.

16. Return pan to oven and bake for 8-10 minutes, until cookies are deep golden brown.

17. They will be slightly puffy and yield a little when with pressed with a finger.

18. Set pan on wire baking rack and run knife through cuts.

19. Cool completely.

20. Run knife through cuts again to make sure cookies are completely separated and lift from pan.

21. ANZAC Cookies will keep in airtight container for 1 week

Maple Cayenne Pecans

Preparation time

50 minutes

Ingredients

- 1 tsp. coconut oil (or other oil, like olive or walnut oil)

- 1 cup raw pecan halves

- 1 Tbsp. pure maple syrup

- 1/8 tsp. cinnamon

- 1/4 tsp. Himalayan sea salt (or regular salt)

- 1/8 tsp. cayenne

Instructions

1. Preheat oven to 325 degrees F.

2. Grease pan lightly with oil. In a medium bowl, combine all other ingredients.

3. Spread pecans evenly on baking sheet.

4. Bake for 15 minutes, stirring every 5 minutes.

5. Remove sheet from oven and transfer to a platter or plate, allowing the pecans to cool fully for 30 minutes before eating.

Red Beet Smoothie Bowl

Preparation time

5 minutes

Ingredients

- 1 cup frozen or fresh berries

- 1/2 cup raw red beets, diced small {approximately 1 medium sized be

- 1 cup Organic Plain Whole Milk Kefir

- 1 banana

- 1/4 cup ground flax

Instructions

1. Blend all of the ingredients until smooth.

2. Top with additional garnishes.

Carrot Cake Smoothie

Preparation time

5 minutes

Ingredients

- 1 frozen banana

- 2 small organic carrots

- 2 tblsp organic chia seeds

- 1/4 cup organic rolled oats

- Splash of preferred milk

- 2 tbls organic yogurt

- Pinch of shredded coconut

- 1 tsp ground cinnamon

- 2 Pecans or walnuts

Optional Ingredients:

- 1 tsp maca powder

- 1-2 medjool dates

Instructions

1.	Blend all of the ingredients minus the coconut, cinnamon, pecans & 1 tablespoon vanilla yoghurt, until smooth.

2.   Pour into a jar and top with remaining tablespoon of yoghurt and sprinkle with cinnamon, shredded coconut and pecans.

3. Enjoy!